Handbook Of Perioperative Care Of Adult Diabetes Patients

OrangeBooks Publication

Smriti Nagar, Bhilai, Chhattisgarh - 490020

Website: **www.orangebooks.in**

First Edition, 2022

ISBN: 978-93-5621-061-5

HANDBOOK OF PERIOPERATIVE CARE OF ADULT DIABETES PATIENTS

DIABETES CARE – BEFORE, DURING AND AFTER SURGERY

Dr VISHWANATH R HIREMATH

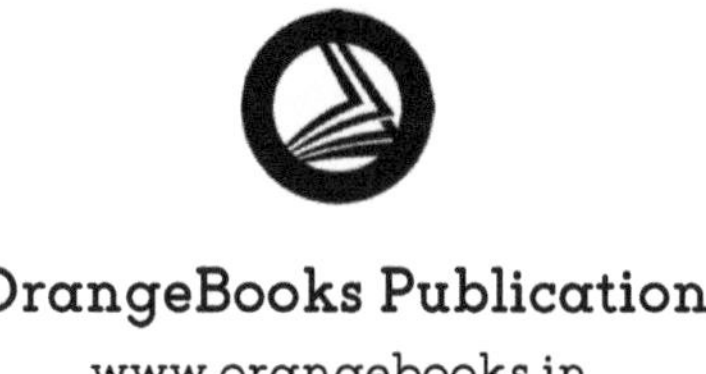

OrangeBooks Publication

www.orangebooks.in

FOREWORD

Dr Harsoor SS
Professor and HOD
Anesthesiology and critical care
Ambedkar Medical College, Bengaluru
Former Director Medical Education
Govt of Karnataka
Past National President Indian Society of India (ISA)

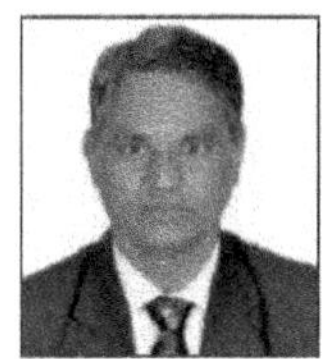

I am indeed honored to write forward for the book **The Handbook of Perioperative Care of Adult Diabetes Mellitus Patients,** authored by Dr. Vishwanath Hiremath. The popular saying of "Diabetes is not a disease, but Mother of all diseases" is more relevant in the Indian context, especially when India is labelled as the Diabetic capital of the World. The author while focussing on the importance of basic pathophysiology and clinical management of Diabetic patients, has laid special emphasis on optimal perioperative care of such patients. All the health care personnel involved in managing the surgical and intensive care of such diabetic patients will be greatly benefitted from this Handbook. The book emphasizes on the evidence-based perioperative care rendered by Anesthesiologists, Postgraduate residents, and Anesthesia technicians, thus making it extremely useful for day-to-day practice. I congratulate the author for making efforts to bring out such a useful book and wish him good luck in future endeavors.

FOREWORD

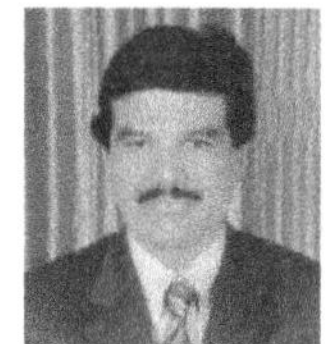

Dr K A Sudharshana Murthy
Former Professor and Head,
Department of Medicine,
JSS Academy of Higher Education &
Research, Mysore.

Type 2 Diabetes Mellitus has assumed epidemic proportions all over the world. India has emerged as the world capital of Diabetes. With the ever-increasing prevalence of Diabetes, its complications and associated diseases are posing therapeutic challenges to the healthcare professional who are involved in the management. Diabetic patients undergoing elective or emergency surgeries have a high risk of developing complications. Appropriate management of diabetes in the pre-operative, intra-operative, and postoperative periods is the key to a successful outcome. The role of anesthesiologists in the management of surgical patients with Diabetes Mellitus is very crucial. Diabetes Mellitus being a metabolic disorder, Anesthesiologists need to have an in-depth knowledge of various complications that could result due to acute stressful condition of surgery involving glucose metabolism and associated electrolyte abnormalities. The management involves achieving a balance between hypoglycemia and hyperglycemia along with correction of other metabolic complications like Ketosis and dyselectrolytemia.

Prof Vishwanath Hiremath has put a lot of effort to simplify the management guidelines of Diabetes Mellitus in surgical patients at various phases of surgery. His academic experience of more than four decades in the field has made this book special, especially for those who are involved in the management of Diabetes Mellitus in surgical patients. I am sure this book, **The Handbook of Perioperative Care of Adult Diabetes Mellitus Patients** will be a ready reckoner, especially for the young practicing anesthesiologists. The chapter wise categorization makes it easy for reference. Information about pathophysiology and metabolic abnormalities of the disease is useful to understand the development of acute complications during surgery and scientific management of the same. I congratulate Prof Hiremath for this effort and wish him good.

PREFACE

With the increase in the prevalence of Diabetes Mellitus (DM); an increasing number of people with diabetes undergo surgery every year. Diabetes is a chronic metabolic disorder with more and more health problems related to the long-term consequences, along with comorbidity, hypertension. Further, the prior condition of pre-diabetic state may exist in the patient for years without overt diabetes. Such an asymptomatic condition is a difficult situation, and challenging to both; patients and treating physicians.

In the long run, diabetic patients land up with vascular and cardiac complications and may get hospitalized for various operative procedures.

This book is penned to familiarize perioperative Physicians i.e., Anesthesia residents, and practicing anesthesiologists in the pathophysiology of stress hyperglycemia, the role of various anti-diabetic medications, optimal glycemic control with targets.

This book covers the in-depth importance of history taking, glycated hemoglobin A1c and antihyperglycemic drugs (oral, noninsulin, and insulin), the significance of optimal glycemic targets in the perioperative period, and the importance of a multidisciplinary professional team approach to enhance the delivery of care to patients in the perioperative period. The purpose of this book will be served if service providers undertake the management of the deserving patients efficiently without hesitation.

Author:
Dr. Vishwanath R Hiremath,
Prof and Head of the Department,
Anesthesiology, SLIMS, Puducherry 605502.

ACKNOWLEDGEMENT

I wish to express my sincere thanks and gratitude to Dr. SS Harsoor, Professor and HOD Anesthesiology, Ambedkar Medical College Bangalore, Ex-President ISA National, Former Director of Medical Education Karnataka for his valuable suggestions. I extend my special thanks and gratitude to Dr. Sudarshan Murthy former Professor and HOD Medicine JSS Medical College Mysore for his scholarly input. I am delighted to thank Dr. S Rajashekharan Director, SLIMS Puducherry, for his constant support and encouragement in bringing this book. Manuscripts have been evaluated by my colleagues and some valuable suggestions have been made, which are incorporated in the text accordingly. I thank Dr. A. Anusha, Dr. Abi Meenashy, and Dr. Sankar Narayanan, my Anesthesia faculties for their contributions in preparing the manuscript. Last but not least I would like to thank M/s Orange Books Publications (P) Ltd , Smriti Nagar, Bhilai, Chhattisgarh for publishing and printing this book.

Dr. Vishwanath R Hiremath,

MD (Anaes)., FICA., FIMSA., PG DIP(DIAB)

ABBREVIATIONS

ACR	Albumin-To-Creatinine Ratio
ADA	American Diabetes Association
BG	Blood glucose
BNP	Brain Natriuretic Peptide
BSL	Blood Sugar Level
CAN	Cardiac Autonomic Neuropathy
DM	Diabetes Mellitus
DPP4	Dipeptidyl peptidase 4
GLP-1	Glucagon-Like Peptide 1
GDM	Gestational Diabetes Mellitus
HbA1c	Glycosylated Hemoglobin
HDC	High Dependency Care
HF	Heart Failure
IFG	Impaired Fasting Glucose
IGT	Impaired Glucose Tolerance
ICU	Intensive Care Unit
IU	International Unit(S)
IV	Intravenous

IVII	Intravenous Insulin Infusion
MMA	Multimodal Analgesia
OHD	Oral Hypoglycemic Drug
PACU	Post-Anesthesia Care Unit
PPV	Pulse Pressure Variation
SGLT2	Sodium-glucose co-transport protein 2
SC	Subcutaneous
SVV	Stroke Volume Variation
T1D	Type 1 Diabetes
T2D	Type 2 Diabetes

CONTENTS

1

Introduction

Diabetes mellitus (DM) is a chronic metabolic disorder, characterized by hyperglycemia due to defects in insulin secretion, insulin action, or a combination of both[1]. India is considered to be the capital of Diabetes. There are about 74.96 million cases of DM in India. Diabetes exists in both rural and urban populations[2]. Nearly 25% of the population having diabetes, may not be aware of the disease until they develop the complications of DM or accidental detection of the condition during the routine health checkup. The prevalence of DM in hospitalized patients is nearly 12-25%[3]. Despite advances in management, many diabetes patients suffer from macrovascular and microvascular complications due to disease, which necessitates more surgical intervention than those without. The presence of an existing or impaired diabetes state increases the perioperative risks due to physiological stress of surgery, anesthetic drugs, fasting state, associated treatment, and infusions with significant morbidity, mortality, and healthcare costs.[4-6]

Hence, patients need optimal glycemic control in all three phases: preoperative, intraoperative, and postoperative period for a safe outcome. Patients need evaluation and optimization by a multidisciplinary team comprising: primary care physician, endocrinologist, ophthalmologist, cardiologist, operating surgeon, and anesthesiologist[7].

Surgery in DM patients is a complicated task. The stress of surgery, anesthesia and acute illness alter homeostasis and lead to stress hyperglycemia. Stress hyperglycemia leads to increased secretion of counter-regulatory hormones; cortisol, glucagon, growth hormone, and epinephrine (catecholamines). Epinephrine stimulates the secretion of glucagon from alpha cells while inhibiting insulin secretion from pancreatic beta cells[8]. Increased levels of stress hormones lead to enhanced lipolysis resulting in high free fatty acid (FFA)levels. Increased FFA leads to insulin resistance and inhibits glucose uptake in skeletal muscle by limiting the intracellular signaling cascade responsible for glucose transport activity. Hyperglycemia also leads to the release of pro-inflammatory cytokines like; tumor necrosis factor-alpha, interleukin 6 (IL6), interleukin 1(IL1), and interleukin 1β leading to infection and sepsis. In addition, hyperglycemia affects both the quantity and quality of leukocytes; their function, phagocytosis, chemotaxis, leading to infection and sepsis. Oxidative stress releases reactive oxygen species and results in direct cellular damage, with vascular and immune dysfunction.[9].

Tight glycemic control in the perioperative period; ongoing treatment (OHA with /or Insulin), NPO (with prolonged fasting) may result in life-threatening hypoglycemia leading to extended hospital and ICU stay and mortality. Hence, the anesthesiologist has an important role in avoiding morbidity and mortality. Even though tight glycemic control is increasingly recognized as a better option in surgical patients there is a paucity of literature regarding overall consensus on the issue[10].

Hence, preoperative glucose optimization, early identification and management of hyper or hypoglycemia, and electrolyte imbalance play a key role in the perioperative care of DM patients undergoing surgery[11].

REFERENCES

1. American Diabetes Association. Diagnosis and classification of diabetes mellitus. Diabetes Care 2017;40(Suppl. 1): S11–24.

2. Kumar A, Goel MK, Jain RB, Khanna P, Chaudhary V. India towards diabetes control: Key issues. Australas Med J. 2013;6(10):524–31.

3. Kaveeshwar SA, Cornwall J. The current state of diabetes mellitus in India. AMJ 2014, 7, 1, 45-48. http//dx.doi.org/10.4066/AMJ.2014.1979.

4. J. E. Shaw, R. A. Sicree, and P. Z. Zimmet, "Global estimates of the prevalence of diabetes for 2010 and 2030," Diabetes Research and Clinical Practice, vol. 87, no. 1, pp. 4–14, 2010.

5. National Diabetes Education Program. Centers for Disease Control and Prevention. Accessed on 11 Mar. 2022. http://ndep.nih.gov/

6. Authoritative Institute of Health and Welfare (AIHW). National health priority areas. 2013. Accessed on 11 Mar. 2022. http://www.aihw.gov.au/national-health-priority-areas/

7. Ljungqvist O, Nygren J, Thorell A. Insulin resistance and elective surgery. Surgery 2000; 128:757–60.

8. Wall RT. Endocrine diseases. In: Hines RL, Marschall SE. 2008. Stoelting's and Anesthesia and Co-existing Disease. 5th ed. Churchill Livingstone; 402-405.

9. Hall GM, Hunter JM, Cooper MS. 2010. Core Topics in Endocrinology in Anesthesia and Critical Care. New York, Cambridge University Press; 7:75-82. 33.

10. Daneman D. 2006. Type I Diabetes. Lancet; 367: 847-58.

11. Bonnie G, Tahseen AC. New guideline on the perioperative management of diabetes- Royal College of Physicians. Clin Med January 202

2

Diagnostic Criteria For Diabetes

a) *Fasting plasma glucose level equal to or greater than 126mg/dL (fasting is defined as no caloric intake for at least 8 hours).*[1]

b) *Random plasma blood glucose level (RBS), equal to or greater than 200mg/dL inpatient with classical symptoms of hyperglycemia; polyuria, polyphagia, and polydipsia1.*

c) *Plasma blood glucose level equal to or greater than 200mg/dL measured two hours after a glucose load of 75g in an oral glucose tolerance test (OGTT)*[1].

d) *Hemoglobin A1C equal to or greater than 6.5%*[1].

Classification of Diabetes Mellitus:
Diabetes is classified in the following categories[2,3]

- Type 1 diabetes
Due to autoimmune β-cell destruction, usually leading to absolute insulin deficiency

- Type 2 diabetes
Due to a progressive loss of β-cell insulin secretion frequently on the background of insulin resistance

- Gestational diabetes mellitus (GDM)

Diabetes diagnosed in the second or third trimester of pregnancy –no overt diabetes before gestation

- Other specific types:

In addition, Hyperglycemia with Diabetes picture may be seen in other conditions like;

   o Monogenic diabetes syndromes

   o Neonatal diabetes

      Maturity-onset diabetes of the young [MODY]

   o Diseases of the exocrine pancreas
      Cystic fibrosis

      Pancreatitis

   o Drug- or chemical induced diabetes
      Glucocorticoid use, treatment of HIV/AIDS, organ transplantation.

      Such patients also require optimal control of BSL while undergoing hospital treatment.

REFERENCES

1. American Diabetes Association. Diagnosis and classification of diabetes mellitus. Diabetes Care 2010;33 (Suppl 1): S62–9.

2. Palermo NE, Gianchandani RY, McDonnell ME, Alexanian SM. Stress hyperglycemia during surgery and anesthesia: pathogenesis and clinical implications. Curr Diab Rep 2016;16:33.

3. Expert Committee on the Diagnosis and Classification of Diabetes Mellitus Report of the Expert Committee on the Diagnosis and Classification of Diabetes Mellitus. Diabetes Care 1997; 20: 1183– 1197.

3

Pathophysiology Of Diabetes Mellitus

DM is a metabolic disorder characterized by hyperglycemia resulting from defects either in insulin secretion (minimal or absolute lack of insulin), or insulin resistance, sometimes both. The chronic hyperglycemia of diabetes leads to long-term complications of macrovascular and microvascular damages leading to destruction, dysfunction, and failure of various organs; especially the eyes, kidneys, nerves, heart, and blood vessels[1].

The deficient action of insulin at the tissue level leads to metabolic abnormalities of carbohydrates, fat, and protein. Occasionally, impaired insulin secretion and defects in insulin action may coexist in the particular patient. However, it may be unclear which abnormality is the primary cause of hyperglycemia[2].

Symptoms of marked hyperglycemia include polyuria, polydipsia, polyphagia, weight loss, and blurred vision. Acute, life-threatening consequences of uncontrolled diabetes are hyperglycemia with ketoacidosis or hyperglycemic hyperosmolar syndrome (HHS)[3].

Long-term complications of DM due to hyperglycemia include microvascular complications like; retinopathy, nephropathy, and peripheral neuropathy and macrovascular complications; atherosclerotic cardiovascular, cerebrovascular, and peripheral arterial diseases[2,4].

The natural course of type-II diabetes mellitus

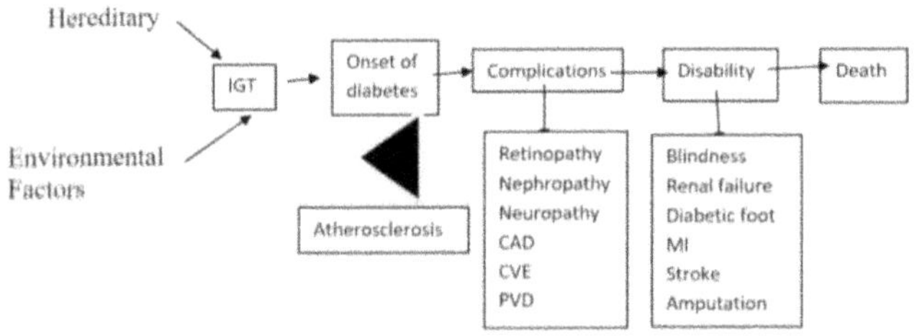

REFERENCES

1. Stumvoll M., Goldstein B.J., van Haeften T.W. Type 2 diabetes: Principles of pathogenesis and therapy. Lancet. 2005; 365:1333–1346. DOI: 10.1016/S0140-6736(05)61032-X.

2. American Diabetes Association. Microvascular complications and foot care: Standards of medical care in diabetes—2018. Diabetes Care. 2018;41: S105–18.

3. Galicia-Garcia U., Benito-Vicente A., Jabari S., Larrea-Sebal A., Siddiqi H., Uribe K.B., Ostolaza H., Martin C. Pathophysiology of Type 2 Diabetes Mellitus. Int. J. Mol. Sci. 2020; 21:6275. DOI: 10.3390/ijms21176275.

4. Pendsey. Practical Management of Diabetes. 2nd edition. New Delhi; St. Louis, Mo.: Jaypee Brothers Medical Publishers Private Limited; 2004. 347p.

4

Stress Hyperglycemia

During the fasting state, usually, normal subjects maintain plasma glucose levels between 80 and 100 mg/dl. The stress of surgery, anesthesia and acute illness alter the balance of hepatic glucose production and glucose utilization in peripheral tissues[1].

An increase in the secretion of counter-regulatory hormones; catecholamines, cortisol, glucagon, and growth hormone result in excessive release of inflammatory cytokines; tumor necrosis factor-α, interleukin-6, and interleukin-1β. Cortisol increases hepatic glucose production, stimulates catabolism, and promotes gluconeogenesis, resulting in elevated BSL. Surging catecholamine, increase glucagon secretion and inhibit the release of insulin by pancreatic β cells. Additionally, the increase in stress hormones leads to enhanced lipolysis (ketogenesis), and high FFA concentrations[2]. FFA inhibits the intracellular signaling cascade in skeletal muscle, glucose transport activity also interferes with the synthesis and/or translocation of the glucose transporter-4 receptor thereby reducing glucose uptake in peripheral tissues. Various such mechanisms result in an altered state of insulin action, leading to a relative state of insulin resistance, that is most pronounced on the first postoperative day and may persist for 9 to 21 days following surgery[3].

Stress hyperglycemia is known to occur in the perioperative period of a few hospitalized patients even without DM. Stress hyperglycemia itself may result in increased risk and adverse outcomes in the admitted patients irrespective of the diabetes status. Hyperglycemia leads to a high infection rate especially nosocomial infections, surgical site infections, and sepsis.

Invariably, hypertension is associated with morbidity with impaired lipid metabolism (dyslipidemia) in patients with diabetes. In the ongoing disease process, the degree of hyperglycemia significantly affects the functions of various organs even without clinical symptoms of DM, for a long period even before DM is detected. During this asymptomatic period, it is possible to demonstrate an abnormality in carbohydrate metabolism by measuring plasma glucose in the fasting state or after a challenge with an oral glucose load or by HbA1C[4]. Preoperative glycemic control results in better outcomes in hospitalized patients. However, severe hypoglycemia with adverse outcomes has been reported in some studies with tight glycemic control. Hypoglycemia is more dangerous than hyperglycemia and should be avoided in the perioperative period for a safe outcome following surgery. The impact of surgery, fasting, and interruptions of routine therapy all contribute to poor glycemic control leading to increased morbidity, mortality, hospital stay, and healthcare cost to DM patients undergoing surgery.

REFERENCES

1. Marik P.E., Bellomo R. Stress hyperglycemia: an essential survival response! *Crit. Care.* 2013;17(2):305.

2. Dungan K, Braithwaite SS, Preiser JC. Stress hyperglycemia. *Lancet.* 2009; 373:1798–1807. DOI: 10.1016/S0140-6736(09)60553-5.

3. Dungan KM, Braithwaite SS, Preiser JC. Stress hyperglycemia. *The Lancet.* 2009;373(9677):1798-1807.

4. Capes SE, Hunt D, Malmberg K, Gerstein HC. Stress hyperglycemia and increased risk of death after myocardial infarction in patients with and without diabetes: a systematic overview. *Lancet.* 2000; 355:773–778. DOI: 10.1016/S0140-6736(99)08415-9.

5

Assessing Glycemic Control

Various studies show a clear association between perioperative hyperglycemia and adverse clinical outcomes. The risk of postoperative complications leading to increased morbidity/ mortality in hospitalized patients has a direct link to the severity of hyperglycemia and long-term BSL control at the time of admission. As such, there is a 50% increase in morbidity and mortality in patients with diabetes compared to patients without the disease[1]. Pathophysiologic changes that occur in the hyperglycemic state significantly contribute to poor outcomes in DM patients. Elevated blood glucose (BG) levels impair neutrophil function, decreased nitric oxide synthase, overproduction of reactive oxygen species, free fatty acids (FFA), and inflammatory mediators. These pathophysiologic changes result in cellular apoptosis, vascular injury (endothelial injury), and immune dysfunctions. Correction of hyperglycemia with insulin administration reduces hospital complications and decreases mortality in operated patients. However, optimal glucose management during the perioperative period is still a subject of debate. Recent randomized controlled trials targeting conventional targets for glycemic control have not demonstrated the significant risk of hyperglycemia, documented in the previous studies[2]. The pendulum of inpatient care has since moved toward more moderate and individualized glycemic targets.

Hyperglycemia is a risk factor for postoperative infections like pneumonia, sepsis, urinary tract infection, acute renal failure, endothelial dysfunction, cerebral ischemia, acute myocardial ischemia/infarction, and impaired healing. Further, the stress response may lead to diabetic adverse events including; diabetic ketoacidosis (DKA) or hyperglycemic hyperosmolar syndrome (HHS) during surgery or in the postoperative period.

Hypokalemia is an associated complication of diabetic ketoacidosis treated with insulin. Insulin drives extracellular potassium ions for intracellular hydrogen ions. Additional loss of potassium in urine due to osmotic diuresis results in hypokalemia. The condition may be complicated with other abnormalities like hypocalcemia, hypomagnesemia, and QT prolongation leading to life-threatening arrhythmias.

Tight glycemic control with insulin may lead to severe life-threatening hypoglycemia in the postoperative period compared to liberal glucose targets[3]. Symptoms of hypoglycemia include tremors, sweating, dizziness, lightheadedness, seizures, and loss of consciousness. Intraoperative hypoglycemia may delay emergence from anesthesia until exogenous glucose is administered to normalize blood sugar.

Careful management of glucose levels in DM patients undergoing major surgeries, including cardiac and orthopedic procedures may minimize the complications, with overall better outcomes. Hospitalized diabetics generally tend to be older, less active, with their glycemic levels being less aggressively controlled. Diabetics undergo certain procedures and surgeries more frequently than nondiabetics and are prone to increased morbidity and mortality[4]. Sometimes unrecognized hypoglycemia results in neuroglycopenia leading to somnolence, unconsciousness, seizures, irreversible neurological insult, and death. Under general anesthesia or deep sedation, neurological manifestations of hypoglycemia may go undetected, leaving the hypoglycemic state unrecognized for a considerable period before initiation of proper management. In general, complications from surgical wounds are more in diabetics. Clinicians must remain alert to identify glucose intolerance, insulin resistance, and associated diabetic pathologies to prevent morbidity and avoid mortality in DM patients. By careful glycemic control strategies, outcome measures of surgery in DM could be at par with nondiabetic patients.

REFERENCES

1. Umpierrez GE, Isaacs SD, Bazargan N, You X, Thaler LM, Kitabchi AE. Hyperglycemia: an independent marker of in-hospital mortality in patients with undiagnosed diabetes. J Clin Endocrinol Metab. 2002;87(3):978–982.

2. Frisch A, Chandra P, Smiley D, Peng L, Rizzo M, Gatfcliffe C, Hudson M, Mendoza J, Johnson R, Lin E, Umpierrez G. Prevalence and clinical outcome of hyperglycemia in the perioperative period in noncardiac surgery. Diabetes Care. 2010;33(8):1783–1788.

3. Kotagal M, Symons RG, Hirsch IB, Umpierrez GE, Farrokhi ET, Flum DR, SCOAP-Certain Collaborative Perioperative hyperglycemia and risk of adverse events among patients with and without diabetes. Ann Surg. 2015;261(1):97–103.

4. Kwon S, Thompson R, Dellinger P, Yanez D, Farrohki E, Flum D. Importance of perioperative glycemic control in general surgery: a report from the Surgical Care and Outcomes Assessment Program. Ann Surg. 2013 Jan;257(1):8

6

Management Of Diabetes Mellitus

Principles of management:

- The first step in diabetes management is lifestyle modification for three months which includes a variety of options like regular exercise (30 minutes per day), yoga, optimization of body weight, less carbohydrate diet, and high protein diet.

- The target HbA1C for a diabetic patient is 6.5. So, if the HbA1c of the patient is more than 7, then always start with oral hypoglycemic agents[1].

- If HbA1c is more than 9 or if blood sugar levels are not controlled with OHA, then always go for insulin[2].

Oral Hypoglycemic Agents (OHA)

There are many classes of OHA which include[1-3]

- Biguanides
- Sulfonylureas
- Meglitinides
- Thiazolidinediones
- Alpha-glucosidase inhibitors
- Glucagon-like peptide-1(GLP-1) receptor agonists
- Dipeptidyl peptidase 4 (DPP-4) inhibitors

- Sodium-glucose cotransport protein 2 (SGLT-2) inhibitors

Biguanide

Metformin is an oral biguanide. It is often used as an OHA to prevent hyperglycemia in patients with type 2 diabetes. It inhibits glucose production in the liver and the incidence of hypoglycemia is less. It should not be prescribed for patients with impaired tissue perfusion, acute kidney injury, gastrointestinal intolerance, or acute hepatic disease. Metformin reduces blood glucose levels by 1-2%. It is usually initiated with a low dose of 500mg once daily, then gradually depending upon the tolerability and response, it is increased to achieve the target blood sugar level. The maximum dose of metformin is 2gm/day The most common side effects are nausea, vomiting, anorexia, diarrhea, vitamin B12 deficiency, and a very rare but serious side-effect is lactic acidosis[1-3].

Sulfonylureas

Successful management of glucose control with sulfonylureas requires some beta cell function.

- ✓ First-generation agents- chlorpropamide, tolazamide, and tolbutamide are outdated nowadays.

- ✓ Second-generation agents - glipizide, glimepiride, and glyburide 1-3.

Second-generation sulfonylureas are preferred over first-generation agents because they are proven to be more potent, with the safest profile being that of glimepiride[4].

Sulfonylureas are contraindicated in patients with hepatic and renal diseases and are also contraindicated in pregnant patients due to the possible prolonged hypoglycemic effect on infants[4].

Meglitinides

Meglitinides, like repaglinide and nateglinide, are secretagogues, Meglitinide shares the same mechanism as that of sulfonylureas; it also binds to the sulfonylurea receptor in β-cells of the pancreas. However, the binding of meglitinide to the receptor is weaker than sulfonylurea[5].

Thiazolidinediones

Rosiglitazone and pioglitazone are agonists of peroxisome proliferator-activated receptors (PPAR) and facilitate increased glucose uptake in numerous tissues including adipose, muscle, and liver[6]. However, there are high concerns about risks overcoming the benefits. Combined insulin- Thiazolidinediones therapy causes heart failure.

GLP-1 Receptor Agonists

The currently GLP-1 receptor agonists available are exenatide and liraglutide. These drugs exhibit increased resistance to enzymatic degradation by Dipeptidyl peptidase 4 (DPP4). GLP-1 analogs are contraindicated in renal failure[6].

DPP-4 Inhibitors

DPP4 inhibitors: Sitagliptin, saxagliptin, vildagliptin and linagliptin are used as a single therapy, or in combination with metformin, and/or a sulfonylurea. The gliptins have not been reported to cause a higher incidence of hypoglycemic events.

SGLT2 Inhibitors

Sodium-glucose cotransporter inhibitors are canagliflozin, dapagliflozin, and empagliflozin. They cause insulin-independent glucose lowering by blocking glucose reabsorption in the proximal renal tubule by inhibiting SGLT2. [7-10]

Insulin

If non-insulin monotherapy like metformin at the maximum tolerated dose (2grams) does not achieve or maintain the HbA1C target over 3 months, then a second oral agent will be added to the regimen. If the HbA1C still remains high a GLP-1 receptor agonist or basal insulin therapy is introduced[1-3]. Insulin therapy (with or without additional agents) is also introduced in patients with newly identified T2DM with severely elevated blood glucose levels > 300-350 mg/dl or HbA1C >10-12%[11].

Basal insulin is the initial insulin regimen, beginning at 10 U or 0.1–0.2 U/kg, depending on the severity of hyperglycemia (titrated by 2–3 U every 4–7 days till the glycemic goal is achieved). Use of basal insulin greater than 0.5 U/kg indicates the need for use of an additional agent[3].

NPH (neutral protamine Hagedorn) insulin carries a low risk of hypoglycemia in individuals without any significant history and it is cheaper.

If basal insulin contributes to acceptable fasting blood glucose, but HbA1C persistently remains above target, then mealtime insulin may be added.

Rapid-acting insulin analog (lispro, aspart, or glulisine) may be used and administered just before meals as a bolus dose.

Sometimes, *bolus insulin* needs to be administered in addition to basal insulin. Rapid-acting analogs are used as bolus formulations due to their prompt onset of action. An insulin pump (continuous subcutaneous insulin infusion) may be used instead, to avoid multiple injections. An ideal insulin regimen should mimic physiological insulin release while providing optimal glycemic control with a low risk of hypoglycemia, weight gain, and fewer daily injections[12].

Insulin drives potassium into the cell and can cause hypokalemia. Components of insulin preparation have the potential to cause allergy. Insulin injections, along with the use of other drugs like TZDs, can precipitate cardiac failure[2,12].

Anesthetic implications of glucose-lowering regimen:

The continuation of the drugs depend upon:
- Type of diabetes
- Nature and extent of the surgical procedure
- Length of pre-and post-operative fasting that is anticipated

- The frequency and daily dosage of medications the patient is taking
- Metabolic state of the patient

Regarding metformin, it is usually stopped 24 hours before surgery and started as soon as the normal diet is resumed only after evaluating renal function tests. However, according to the JBDS (Joint British Diabetes Society) Association, if the patient posted for operation is anticipated to skip only one meal i.e., a short starvation period, then he can continue taking Metformin on the day of surgery also.

If the patient is diagnosed with some renal dysfunction during the pre-operative evaluation, then metformin should be discontinued for such patient (until renal function normalizes) and switched over to some other OHA.

It is generally recommended that sulfonylurea and insulin-secretagogues be discontinued on the day of surgery, only to avoid the risk of hypoglycemia.

Patients on SGLT-2 inhibitors should be advised to stop their medication 24 hours prior to surgery. It is a safety measure because studies have reported an increased incidence of DKA with SGLT-2 inhibitors.

DPP-4 inhibitors have good glycemic control without the risk of hypoglycemia. Hence, they can be continued on the day of surgery.

With regard to insulin:

The night before surgery: long-acting insulin (basal insulin) should be reduced to 75-80% of the usual dose and rapid-acting insulin can be given at their usual dose.

On the morning of surgery: long-acting insulin can be given at 50% of their usual dose and rapid-acting insulin can be withheld.[13]

Table 1: Medications in the peri-operative period[13]

OHA	Day before surgery	Day of surgery (minimally invasive surgery/ normal intake is anticipated on the same day)	Day of surgery (extensive surgery/ NPO is expected to be prolonged/ anticipated fluid shifts or HD changes)
Secretagogues	Take	Hold	Hold
SGLT-2 inhibitors	Hold	Hold	Hold
Thiazolidinediones	Take	Take	Hold
Metformin	Take*	Take*	Hold
DPP-4 inhibitors	Take	Take	Take

*Hold if patient having a procedure with intravenous contrast dye administration, particularly in those with GFR<45ml/min.

DPP- Dipeptidyl peptidase, HD- hemodialysis, SGLT-2 – Sodium Glucose cotransporter-2

REFERENCES

1. American Diabetes Association, "Standards of medical care in diabetes—2014," *Diabetes Care*, vol. 37, supplement 1, pp. S14–S80, 2014.

2. American Diabetes Association. 9. Pharmacologic approaches to glycemic treatment: standards of medical care in diabetes-2021. *Diabetes Care* 2021;44: (Suppl 1): S111–24.

3. Chaudhury A, Dufour C, Reddy Dendi VSR, et al. . Clinical review of antidiabetic drugs: implications for type 2 diabetes mellitus management. *Front Endocrinol (Lausanne)* 2017;8:06.

4. Perks P, Reimann F, Green N, Gribble F, Ashcroft F. Sulfonylurea stimulation of insulin secretion. *Diabetes* (2002) 51(3):5368–76.10.2337/diabetes.51.2007.S368.

5. Internal Clinical Guidelines Team. *Type 2 Diabetes in Adults: Management*. London: National Institute for Health and Care Excellence; (2015). 28 p.

6. Bailey CJ. The current drug treatment landscape for diabetes and perspectives for the future. *Clin Pharmacol Ther* (2015) 98(2):170–84.10.1002/cpt.144.

7. James JC, Andrew SR, Charles FS, Jr, Annie N. PA-C diagnosis and management of diabetes: synopsis of 2016; American Diabetes Association standards of medical care in diabetes. *Ann Intern Med* (2016) 164:542–52.10.7326/M15-3016.

8. Ismail-Beigi F. Pathogenesis and glycemic management of type 2 diabetes mellitus: a physiological approach. *Arch Iran Med* (2012) 15(4):239–46.

9. Stein SA, Lamos EM, Davis SN. A review of the efficacy and safety of oral antidiabetic drugs. *Expert Opin Drug Saf* 2013; 12:153–75.

10. Chaudhury A, Dufour C, Reddy Dendi VSR, et al. Clinical review of antidiabetic drugs: implications for type 2 diabetes mellitus management. *Front Endocrinol (Lausanne)* 2017; 8:06.

11. Wilcox G. Insulin and insulin resistance. *Clin Biochem Rev*. 2005;26(2):19-39.

12. Rahman MS, Hossain KS, Das S, et al. Role of Insulin in Health and Disease: An Update. *Int J Mol Sci*. 2021;22(12):6403. Published 2021 Jun 15. doi:10.3390/ijms22126403.

13. Elizabeth W. Duggan, Karen Carlson, Guillermo E.Umipierrez. Perioperative hyperglycemia management: an update. Anesthesiology 2017;126: 547-560.

7

Metabolic Response To Surgery And Anesthesia

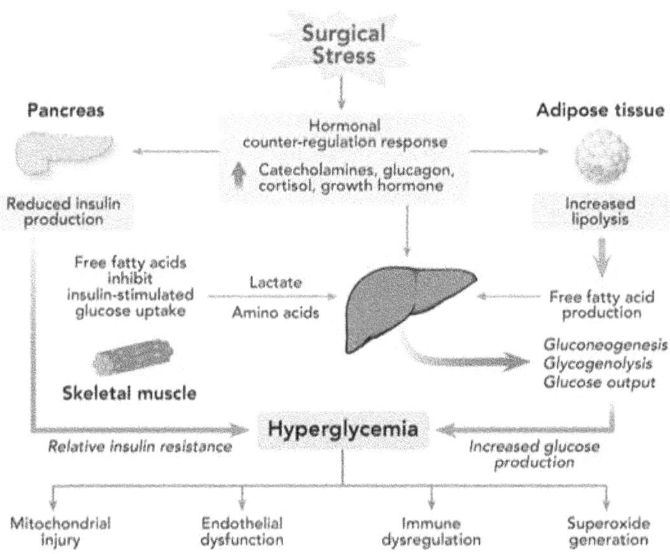

Stress and surgical trauma result in increased production of stress hormones, their magnitude depends on the severity of the surgery and postoperative complications. In diabetic patients, this type of metabolic response results in increased levels of cortisol and catecholamines with reduced insulin sensitivity. The enhanced sympathetic activity also results in reduced insulin secretion with simultaneously increased secretion of growth hormone and glucagon[1-3].

REFERENCES

1. Palermo NE, Gianchandani RY, McDonnell ME, Alexanian SM. Stress Hyperglycemia During Surgery and Anesthesia: Pathogenesis and Clinical Implications. Curr Diab Rep. 2016 Mar;16(3):33.

2. Dagogo-Jack S, Alberti KGMM. Management of diabetes mellitus in surgical patients. *Diabetes Spectrum.* 2002;15(1):44-48.

3. Elizabeth W. Duggan, Karen Carlson, Guillermo E.Umipierrez. Perioperative hyperglycemia management: an update. Anesthesiology 2017;126: 547-560.

8

Pre-Operative Evaluation Of Patients With Dm

Preoperative assessment of the patient involves a comprehensive evaluation, control of metabolic disorder, comorbidities, and management of complications (microvascular and macrovascular) of the disease itself for safe surgical outcome.

History

History involves details regarding:

- Diabetes mellitus – type of diabetes mellitus, current glycemic control, related complications, susceptibility to hypoglycemia -including hypoglycemic unawareness, treatment strategy with OHA regimen, and adherence to the treatment

- Surgery- the type of surgery-daycare, elective, time-sensitive, emergency or urgency, anticipated duration of surgery, and fasting.

- Glycated hemoglobin- A: preoperative hemoglobin A1c (HbA1c) should be checked, if not tested in the preceding three months. There is an association of HbA1c with surgical outcomes. The aim is not to defer the surgery with just HbA1c level, it is recommended to assess glycemic control and recognize the patient with undiagnosed DM. There are no validated HbA1c cut-off values. The level of more than 7.8%, is associated with increased cardiovascular-related morbidity. Elective surgery should be postponed if HbA1c>10%. Emergency and time-sensitive procedures should not be delayed to achieve target HbA1c, instead, the focus should be on optimizing perioperative glucose control[1-3].

Autonomic Dysfunction

Autonomic dysfunction may be detected in 40% of type 1 diabetics. The patient should be evaluated for the typical symptoms and signs of postural hypotension, gastroparesis, gustatory sweating, and nocturnal diarrhea. It is worthwhile to assess all diabetic patients for autonomic neuropathy.[4-8]

a) **Heart Rate Recording**
- Three lead ECG with electrodes on the anterior chest wall
- Reference electrode at the midaxillary line at T4 level
- Tests of heart rate variability measured as R-R interval.

b) **Blood Pressure Recording**
- Continuous or intermittent recording
- Brachial/wrist/finger cuffs used
- Plethysmography and arterial tonometry for noninvasive recording.

Parasympathetic Function Tests:

a) Heart Rate Response to Valsalva Maneuver

Procedure:

- Baseline BP and heart rate measured 3 minutes before the test
- Patient takes deep inhalation, complete exhalation followed by deep inhalation again
- Patient then exhales deeply into a mouthpiece for 15 seconds
- Mouthpiece is connected to a pressure transducer to measure expiratory pressure
- Expiratory pressure maintained at 40 mm Hg
- BP and heart rate measured throughout the maneuver and for 60 seconds after the maneuver
- Average of two trials taken for analysis.

Interpretation
- Valsalva Ratio = Maximum heart rate/ Minimum heart rate
- Normal ratio > 1.21[9].

b) Respiratory Sinus Arrhythmia

Procedure:

- Done with the patient in supine
  Breathing at a rate of 6 breaths/min with slow inspiration and expiration
  This provides maximum heart rate variability
- Six to eight cycles are recorded in one/two trials
- Timed breathing potentiates sinus arrhythmia
- Reduced heart rate variability with respiration is seen with autonomic dysfunction..

c) Heart Rate Response to Standing

- Baseline heart rate measured in the supine position
- Patient asked to stand up quickly
- Heart rate variability measured for at least 1 minute of active standing.
- Interpretation
- 30:15 ratio: HR at 30 seconds of standing / HR at 15 seconds of standing
- Normal ratio > 1.

Sympathetic Function Tests

a) Blood Pressure response to Sustained Hand Grip
- Sustained handgrip measured by a dynamometer
- Blood pressure measured every minute for 5 minutes
- Initial diastolic BP subtracted from DBP just before the release of hand grip
  Normal value >16mmHg.

b) Blood Pressure response to standing

- Patient moves from supine to standing position
- Standing systolic BP subtracted from supine SBP
- Normal value <10mmHg.

Tilt Table Test Procedure
- Patient lies supine on tilt table and belt placed around the waist
- BP and heart rate measured throughout the test
- Baseline BP recorded for at least 3 minutes
- Patient tilted slowly to 60–80° upright angle
- Patient told to report any symptoms
- Patient returned to horizontal supine position
- HR and BP monitored

Interpretation

Normal values:

–Decrease in systolic BP < 20 mm Hg

–Decrease in diastolic BP < 10 mm Hg.[11,12]

c) Sympathetic Skin Response (SSR)

Procedure

- Standard EMG instrument used
- Sweep speed of 10 sec and bandpass filter of 1–2000 Hz used
- Small recording electrode attached to the palmar and dorsal surface of hands and feet
- Stable baseline recorded before administering stimulus (electrical/loud noise)
- Sympathetic Skin Response noted
- Recordings can be obtained simultaneously from hands and feet
- 3–4trials obtained.

Interpretation

- Normal response: Monophasic or biphasic deflection which habituates with time
- Abnormal response: Absent SSR.

Peripheral Neuropathy

The commonest type of peripheral neuropathy is the "glove and stocking" type. Diabetics are also prone to mono neuritis multiplex and some particularly painful sensory neuropathies. Poor patient positioning is more likely to result in pressure sores that are often slow to heal given poor peripheral blood flow. Documentation of existing neuropathy is prudent, especially if considering a regional technique[12].

Cardiovascular

Diabetics are more prone to ischemic heart disease (IHD), hypertension, peripheral vascular disease, cerebrovascular disease, cardiomyopathy, and perioperative myocardial infarction. Ischemia may be "silent" as a result of neuropathy. Routine ECG should be performed and appropriate stress testing if in doubt. The degree of cardiovascular (CV) risk is heterogeneous in the diabetes population, as it is linked to coexisting risk factors such as arterial hypertension, lipid abnormalities, smoking, and familial history of early CV problems, and specific factors such as glycemic control, duration of diabetes and, in particular, the presence of nephropathy. The presence of microalbuminuria is associated with increased CV risk in both T1D and T2D and is greater in the presence of macroproteinuria or renal failure. Age, duration of diabetes, coronary artery disease (CAD), and the presence of albuminuria are all associated with increased risk of HF[6,13].

Cardiovascular autonomic neuropathy (CAN)

Persistent tachycardia, orthostatic hypotension in particular (often iatrogenic in origin), postprandial hypotension, and hypoglycemia unawareness are symptoms of severe CAN. Autonomic neuropathy can result in sudden tachycardia, bradycardia, postural hypotension, and profound hypotension after the central neuraxial blockade. If CAN is detected, drugs that might induce orthostatic hypotension should be avoided; the

QT interval should be measured by standard ECG (at the minimum) and, if prolonged, then a 24-hour ECG recording should be performed to detect ventricular ectopic beats[6,11].

Respiratory

Diabetics, especially the obese and smokers are more prone to respiratory infections and might have abnormal spirometry. Chest physiotherapy, humidified oxygen, and bronchodilators should be considered[6].

Gastrointestinal

Gastroparesis is characterized by a delay in gastric emptying without any gastric outlet obstruction. Increased gastric contents increase the risk of aspiration. Symptoms classically include anorexia, nausea, vomiting, abdominal pain, sensation of bloating, early satiety, and/or slowing of digestion. If clinical signs suggestive of gastroparesis are present, then measurement of the gastric antrum by gastric ultrasound can distinguish whether the stomach is full or not. Gastric ultrasound can also identify any solid residues. If there is any doubt of 'full-stomach', rapid sequence induction intubation of anesthesia should be carried out[6,10.] Always ask about symptoms of reflux and consider a rapid sequence induction with cricoid pressure even in elective procedures. If available prescribe an H2 antagonist such as Ranitidine 150mg plus Metoclopramide 10mg, at least 2 hours preoperatively[6].

Renal

Diabetes is one of the commonest causes of end-stage renal failure. Hyperkalemia and proteinuria are likely to indicate kidney damage. Ensure adequate hydration to reduce postoperative renal dysfunction. The severity of renal disease depends on the urinary albumin-to-creatinine ratio (ACR) and glomerular filtration rate (GFR). It is recommended to test 2-3 urine samples over 6 months to confirm the diagnosis of CKD.[6,14,15]

Immune System

Diabetics are prone to all types of infection. Indeed, an infection might worsen diabetic control. Tight glycemic control will reduce the incidence and severity of infections and is a routine practice in the management of sepsis and diabetic foot infections. All invasive procedures should be performed under strict aseptic precautions[6].

Other:

Autonomic neuropathy predisposes to hypothermia under anesthesia

Diabetics are prone to cataracts and retinopathy. Prevent surges in blood pressure, for example at induction, as this might cause rupture of the new retinal vessels.

Airway Evaluation

All diabetic patients require thorough airway evaluation. Glycosylation of collagen in the cervical and temporomandibular joints can cause difficulty in intubation.

Restricted mobility of upper cervical spines in DM patients may result in difficult tracheal intubation due to stiff joint syndrome (SJS), with disability of neck extension resulting in poor or impossible visualization of glottis opening during direct laryngoscopy. SJS must be assessed preoperatively by performing the "prayer sign". The patient is asked to put his hand in the position for prayer, if stiffening of interphalangeal joints prevents palmer sides of fists to touch each other, the test is positive and predicts difficult intubation.

Predictors of the difficult airway are the same in diabetics as in non-diabetic groups.

Palm Print Sign:
The patient is made to sit; the palm and fingers of the right hand are painted with blue ink, patient then presses the hand firmly against a white paper placed on a hard surface[16,17]

It is categorized as:

- ➤ Grade 0 –All the phalangeal areas are visible.

- ➤ Grade 1 –Deficiency in the interphalangeal areas of the 4th and 5th digits.

- ➤ Grade 2 –Deficiency in interphalangeal areas of 2nd to 5th digits.

- ➤ Grade 3 –Only the tips of digits are seen.

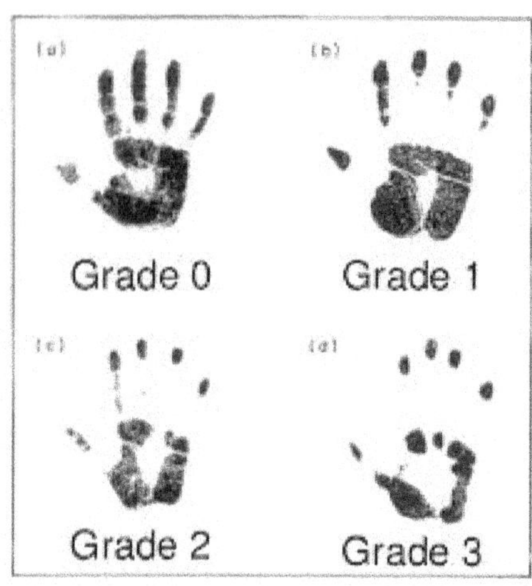

Prayer Sign:

The patient is asked to bring both the palms together as 'Namaste' and the sign is categorized as:[1,2]

> ➢ Positive – When there is a gap between palms.

> ➢ Negative – When there is no gap between palms.

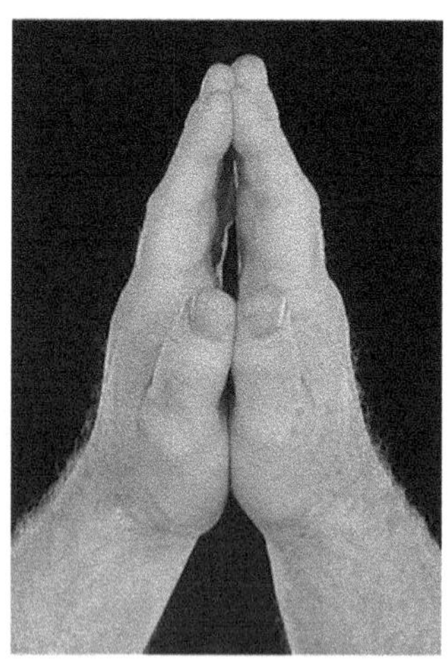

Basic investigations in the pre-operative assessment are:

- Hemoglobin, ESR
- Serum creatinine, BUN (diabetic nephropathy)
- Chest x-ray
- Urine examination for glucose, albumin, and microscopy
- Fasting and post-prandial blood sugars
- Lipid profile including total cholesterol, triglyceride, HDL
- HbA1c (to look for the sugar control over previous 3months)
- Resting ECG
- Thyroid-stimulating hormone (to rule out auto-immune etiology)
- ECHO is done to look for associated cardiomyopathy, ejection fraction, conduction abnormalities, coronary artery disease

REFERENCES

1. Bardia A, Khabbaz K, Mueller A, Mathur P, Novack V, Talmor D, Subramaniam B. The Association Between Preoperative Hemoglobin A1C and Postoperative Glycemic Variability on 30-Day Major Adverse Outcomes Following Isolated Cardiac Valvular Surgery. Anesth Analg. 2017 Jan;124(1):16-22.

2. Dogra P, Jialal I. Diabetic Perioperative Management. [Updated 2021 Sep 28]. In: StatPearls [Internet]. Treasure Island (FL): StatPearls Publishing; 2022 Jan-. Available from: https://www.ncbi.nlm.nih.gov/books/NBK540965/

3. Pendsey. Practical Management of Diabetes. 2nd edition. New Delhi; St. Louis, Mo.: Jaypee Brothers Medical Publishers Private Limited; 2004. 15 p.

4. Marks JB, Hirsch IB. Surgery and diabetes mellitus. In: DeFronzo RA, ed. Current therapy of diabetes mellitus. St. Louis: Mosby, 1998:247–54.

5. Escalante DA, Kim DK, Garber AJ. Atherosclerotic cardiovascular disease. In: DeFronzo RA, ed. Current therapy of diabetes mellitus. St. Louis: Mosby, 1998:176–82.

6. Cosson E, Catargi B, Chaisson G, Jacqueminet S, Ichai C, Leguerrier AM, Ouattara A, Tauveron I, Bismuth E, Benhamou D, Valensi P. Practical management of diabetes patients before, during and after surgery: A joint French diabetology and anaesthesiology position statement. Diabetes Metab. 2018 Jun 1;44(3):200-16.

7. Jothinath, K. Neuroanesthesia. In: Anesthesia Review for DNB Students. India: Jaypee Brothers Medical Publishers Pvt. Limited. 2020. p94-96.

8. Zygmunt A, Stanczyk J. Methods of evaluation of autonomic nervous system function. *Arch Med Sci.* 2010;6(1):11-18. doi:10.5114/aoms.2010.13500

9. Levy N, Dhatariya K. Pre-operative optimization of the surgical patient with diagnosed and undiagnosed diabetes: a practical review. *Anesthesia.* 2019; 74:58-66.

10. Vinik AI, Maser RE, Mitchell BD, Freeman R. Diabetic autonomic neuropathy. Diabetes Care. 2003;26(5):1553-1579.

11. Vinik AI, Ziegler D. Diabetic cardiovascular autonomic neuropathy. Circulation. 2007;115(3):387-397. 3. Harati

Y. Diabetic neuropathies: unanswered questions. Neurol Clin. 2007;25(1):303-317.

12. Bilal N, Erdogan M, Ozbek M, et al. Increasing severity of cardiac autonomic neuropathy is associated with the increasing prevalence of nephropathy, retinopathy, and peripheral neuropathy in Turkish type 2 diabetics. J Diabetes Complications. 2008;22(3):181-185.

13. Low PA. Testing the autonomic nervous system. *Semin Neurol.* 2003; 23:407–21.

14. Carnethon MR, Prineas RJ, Temprosa M, Zhang ZM, Uwaifo G, Molitch ME. Diabetes Prevention Program Research Group. The association among autonomic nervous system function, incident diabctcs, and intervention arm in the Diabetes Prevention Program. *Diabetes Care.* 2006; 29:914–19.

15. Moghissi ES, Korytkowski MT, DiNardo M, et al. American Association of Clinical Endocrinologists and American Diabetes Association consensus statement on inpatient glycemic control. *Diabetes Care.* 2009; 32:1119–1131.

16. Nadal JLY, Fernandez BG, Escobar IC, Black M, Rosenblatt WH. The palm print as a sensitive predictor of difficult laryngoscopy in diabetics. *Acta Anaesthesiologica Scandinavica.* 1998;42(2):199-203.

17. Hashim VK, Thomas M. Sensitivity of palm print sign in the prediction of difficult laryngoscopy in diabetes: a comparison with other airway indices. *Indian J Anaesth.* 2014;58(3):298–302. DOI: 10.4103/0019-5049.135042.

9

Anesthetic Management

Objectives of anesthetic management involve:

- Understanding the history and type of diabetes mellitus, glycated hemoglobin A1c and antihyperglycemic drugs (oral, non-insulin injectables, and insulin) in the preoperative period.
- Insulin management in non-critically and critically ill surgical patients; including dose calculation and transitioning from intravenous to subcutaneous insulin.
- Identify and describe the significance of optimal glycemic control targets in the perioperative period.

To understand effectively we have classified this heading into the pre-operative review, intra-operative and post-operative management.

Pre-operative:

Usually, diabetic patients are to be taken up for surgery first among the list of posted patients. Scheduling of surgery should be aimed at minimizing the nil per oral duration for diabetic patients.

In elective surgery, already optimization would have been done. The fasting blood sugar levels on the day of surgery must be less than 140mg/dl according to ADA guidelines and the plasma or urine ketone on the day of surgery is always done to rule out ketosis. When a patient presents with DKA on the day of surgery, elective surgery is always contraindicated. Postpone elective/ non-urgent surgery if there is an acute increase in glucose>400mg/dl.[1]

For emergency surgery, where optimization is impossible, except in the most pressing surgical circumstances (such as torrential and uncontrolled hemorrhage or the acutely compromised airway), such patients always require full stabilization before anesthesia and surgery can be contemplated. As the blood glucose concentration declines, the acidosis resolves and the serum electrolytes normalize, and the contraindications to anesthesia and surgery diminish. In non-life-threatening surgical situations, the ketoacidosis should be allowed to resolve fully and the patient stabilized on a GIK (Glucose-Insulin-Potassium) regimen infusion before surgery.[2] In the case of patients with pressing surgical problems, such as vascular or intra-abdominal emergencies, the surgeon and anesthesiologist must weigh the risks of delay against those of incomplete correction compounded by the surgical stress response in deciding the optimum time for surgical intervention.

Overall, the decision depends on:

- Patient's stability
- Need for surgery
- Risk of surgery
- Ability of the patient to achieve glucose control if surgery is postponed

Intra-Operative Management:

Daycare surgeries should be considered for diabetic patients whenever possible. Chronic diabetics are usually better at managing their diabetes themselves. And in such patients admitting the patient and in-patient management procedures may disrupt the normal diabetes homeostasis. So day-care surgeries with correct pre-anesthetic instructions are better.

Monitoring includes basic ASA monitors such as ECG, NIBP, Pulse-oximeter. In co-existing cardiac conditions, invasive blood pressure monitoring may be required, in renal disease CVP guided fluid management may be necessary.

Blood glucose needs to be monitored every 1-2 hours in high-risk cases, whereas every 4-6 hours is sufficient for low-risk patients. CBG should be checked at induction and at least hourly if the patient is on insulin or insulin-secretagogues; otherwise, a minimum of 2 hourly CBG is necessary. Immediate access to a glucometer is essential.

In high-risk cases every hour monitoring of blood glucose, arterial pH, electrolytes (especially potassium and phosphate), and fluid monitoring is essential.

Care in positioning a diabetic patient is very important since they are more vulnerable to pressure/ stretch injuries and orbital injury in prone position because of the already compromised state (peripheral vascular disease and peripheral neuropathy). Adequate padding is a must.[3]

In case of a difficult airway (stiff-joint syndrome), awake intubation is preferred. RSI (rapid sequence intubation) is the choice in a diabetic because of the associated gastroparesis and aspiration risk due to autonomic neuropathy).

The fluid of choice in a diabetic will be normal saline and half normal saline. (Although, excess NS infusion can be dangerous leading to hyperchloremic acidosis).

Whenever possible, regional anesthesia techniques (spinal, epidural, nerve blocks) should be preferred over general anesthesia.

In an emergency surgery presenting with DKA, at least partial correction of intravenous volume depletion and electrolyte imbalance (hypokalemia) is necessary to prevent undue cardiac arrhythmia and resistant hypotension.

In elective surgery, with wide fluctuations in blood glucose levels, it is preferable to follow the GIK regimen (500ml of 5%D with 5U insulin and 20mmol of KCl is started at 100ml/hour).[4]

Due to pre-op metabolic derangements, acute insulin resistance, the stress of surgery and anesthesia, there is widespread potential for the development of perioperative hyperglycemia. Hypothermia and hypovolemia are very common in the post-op state thereby making subcutaneous insulin absorption erratic. That's the reason one should always prefer intravenous insulin in the perioperative period.[1]

Although variable-rate insulin infusion (VRII) is usually started the day before surgery and has the advantage of strict glucose control, it also has equal potential and a more devastating risk of hypoglycemia. Use of VRII is adopted preferably in the following scenarios:

- ✓ Emergency surgery

- ✓ Diabetic patients (type-1 and type-2) undergoing surgery, who's anticipated NPO duration is expected to skip more than 1 meal

- ✓ Type-1 diabetics who have not received basal insulin

- ✓ Persistent peri-operative hyperglycemia

- ✓ Suboptimal control (HbA1c more than 8.5%)

The Surviving Sepsis Campaign recommends maintaining glucose levels below 180 mg/dL; the 2014 European Society of Cardiology guidelines for perioperative cardiac management in noncardiac surgery patients do take into account the results of the NICE-SUGAR study and recommend maintaining glucose levels less than 180 mg/dL in postoperative patients. The Society of Thoracic Surgeons (for cardiac surgery) targets 150 to 180 mg/dL, whereas the guidelines from the American College of Physicians recommend keeping glucose below 180 mg/dL in critically ill patients.[5,6] In sharp contrast to the above, van den Berghe et al. study reported a 42% relative reduction in ICU mortality in critically ill surgical patients treated to a target blood glucose of 80 to 110 mg/dL (intensive control) over liberal control (around 180mg/dl).[7]

So it is better to maintain blood sugar level between 110-180mg/dL in the perioperative period, in-order to avoid the complications of hyperglycemia and life-threatening hypoglycemia.

REFERENCES

1. Tuttnauer A, Levin PD, BChir MB. Diabetes Mellitus and Anesthesia. *Anesthesiol Clin.* 2006; 24:579–97.

2. Dhatariya K, Levy N, Kilvert A, et al. NHS Diabetes guideline for the perioperative management of the adult patient with diabetes. *Diabetic Medicine* 2012; **29**: 420–33.

3. Houlden R, Capes S, Clement M, Miller D. In-hospital management of diabetes. *Canadian Journal of Diabetes* 2013; **37**(Suppl 1): S77– 81.

4. McAnulty GR, Robertshaw HJ, Hall GM. Anaesthetic management of patients with diabetes mellitus. *British Journal of Anaesthesia.* 2000;85(1):80-90.

5. Umpierrez G, Cardona S, Pasquel F, Jacobs S, Peng L, Unigwe M, Newton CA, Smiley-Byrd D, Vellanki P, Halkos M, Puskas JD, Guyton RA, Thourani VH. Randomized Controlled Trial of Intensive Versus Conservative Glucose Control in Patients Undergoing Coronary Artery Bypass Graft Surgery: GLUCO-CABG Trial. Diabetes Care. 2015 Sep;38(9):1665-72

6. Griesdale DE, de Souza RJ, van Dam RM, Heyland DK, Cook DJ, Malhotra A, Dhaliwal R, Henderson WR, Chittock DR, Finfer S, Talmor D. Intensive insulin therapy and mortality among critically ill patients: a meta-analysis including NICE-SUGAR study data. *CMA.* 2009;180(8):821–827.

7. Van den Berghe G, Wouters P, Weekers F, et al (2001)
    Intensive insulin therapy in critically ill patients. N Engl J
    Med 345:1359–1367

10

Post-Operative Care And Concern

Depending upon the intraoperative glycemic control, insulin requirement, hemodynamic stability, and anesthetic outcome, patients will be managed in the post-operative care unit or intensive care unit, or high dependency care unit as per the need. The type, duration, and complexity of the surgery are important factors in deciding about the duration of postoperative fasting and resuming insulin therapy.[1,2]

Perioperative targeted blood sugar is recommended in the range of 110-180 mg/dL for the majority of critically ill and non-critically ill patients. This is to avoid hypoglycemia and the complications of hyperglycemia.

Poorly controlled pain is a risk factor for hyperglycemia. Although the usual analgesics in their normal dose range do not affect blood sugar levels, it is still preferable to opt for regional anesthesia whenever possible.

Regarding the changeover from intravenous to subcutaneous insulin, for patients who have started their oral feeds and their sugar levels are almost under control, it is safe to change over to subcutaneous insulin. Some studies say to change over to subcutaneous, provided the blood sugar levels are within the normal range for 24 hours. For patients who have not been on prior insulin therapy, but were only started on insulin perioperatively, it is better to go for subcutaneous insulin post-operatively. For such patients, insulin can be given at a dose of 1 mU/kg/day (half long-acting and half rapid-acting).[1,2]

Blood sugar monitoring should be performed on a routine basis at least in the immediate post-op period to detect not only hyperglycemia but also hypoglycemia.

Thus, care is conditioned by three parameters:
- Type of diabetes
- Prior treatment
- Perioperative glycemic control after minor or major surgery

Based on the type of surgery:
- After recovery in the PACU, ambulatory surgery patients who are stable and tolerating oral intake can be discharged home on the previous antihyperglycemic regimen.
- Non-critically ill patients who require hospitalization are admitted to the surgical/medical ward on subcutaneous (SC) insulin.
  - ✓ In case of poor or no oral intake, basal plus correctional insulin is preferred.
  - ✓ For a patient on oral feeds, the insulin regimen should consist of basal, nutritional, and correctional components

- Critically ill patients should be managed in an intensive care unit with continuous insulin infusion (CII) with regular insulin, with BG monitoring every 1 to 2 hours.[1,2]

REFERENCES

1. Elizabeth W. Duggan, Karen Carlson, Guillermo E.Umipierrez. Perioperative hyperglycemia management: an update. Anesthesiology 2017;126: 547-560.

2. Grant B, Chowdhury TA. New guidance on the perioperative management of diabetes. *Clin Med.* 2022;22(1):41-44.

INDEX

A

ANNEXURE -1

Interpretation of OGTT (oral glucose tolerance test)

	Normal (NOT)	IFG (impaired fasting glucose)	IGT (impaired glucose tolerance)	Diabetes
Fasting value	<110	110-126	110-126	>126
The 2-hours post glucose value	<140	<140	>=140	>200

ADA Diagnostic Criteria for GDM
One step Approach at 24-28 weeks gestation
Plasma glucose measurement is done when the patient is fasting (overnight fast over 8 hours), then a 75gm OGTT is performed, with plasma glucose measurement is done at 1 and 2 hours. The diagnosis of GDM is made when any of the following is met or exceeded

- Fasting: 92 mg/dL

- 1 hour: 180 mg/dL

- 2 hours: 153 mg/dL

Two step Approach at 24-28 weeks gestation

Plasma glucose measurement is done when the patient is fasting (overnight fast over 8 hours), then a 50gm OGTT is performed, and plasma glucose measurement is done at 1 hour. If the plasma glucose level after 1 hour is more than 130 mg/dL, 135 mg/dL, or 140 mg/dL, fasting 100gm OGTT is performed.

The diagnosis of GDM is made if at least two of the following four plasma glucose levels are met or exceeded

- Fasting: 92 mg/dL

- 1 hour: 180 mg/dL

- 2 hours: 153 mg/dL

- 3 hours: 140 mg/dL

ANNEXURE -2

PRE-OPERATIVE INSULIN ADJUSTEMENTS

TYPE OF INSULIN	EVENING PRIOR TO SURGERY	MORNING OF SURGERY
Long-acting insulin##	75-80% of usual dose	75-80% of usual dose
Intermediate acting insulin	Usual dose	50% of usual dose
Premixed insulin	Usual dose	50% of usual dose**
Nutritional Insulin	Usual dose	HOLD

Reduce long-acting insulin by 50-75% in patients who take large components of basal insulin (>60% of TDD), total daily dose of insulin >80 units or prone to hypoglycemia (elderly, advanced renal or hepatic disease, malnourished).

**When feasible, long-acting insulin is preferred over premixed formulation on the morning of surgery, which is usually ¾ of total daily pre-mixed insulin.

CORRECTIONAL INSULIN SCALE

Blood Glucose (mg /dl)	Insulin Sensitive Scale (TDD < 40 units, insulin naive, age > 70 years, renal or hepatic disease)	Insulin Standard Scale	Insulin Resistant Scale (TDD > 80 units, BMI > 35 Kg/m2, on high dose steroids)	Night-time Dosing Scale (at bedtime and 3am)
150 - 199	1	2	3	0
200 - 249	2	4	6	2
250 - 299	3	6	9	3
300 - 349	4	8	12	4
350 - 399	5	10	15	5
≥ 400	CALL PROVIDER FOR BG ≥ 400			

Handbook on Perioperative Care in Adult Diabetic Patients

Dr. Vishwanath R Hiremath

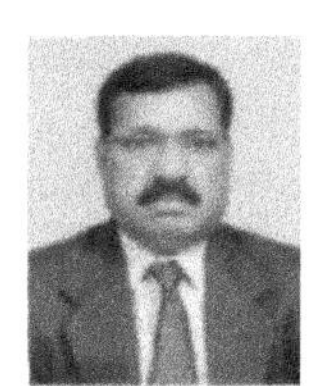

Working as Professor and HOD in the Department of Anesthesiology and Critical care, Sri Lakshmi Narayana Institute of Medical Sciences, Puducherry. Having Graduated from Karnataka Medical College, Hubli, he has done his Post graduation from Grant Medical College / Sir J.J Group of Hospitals, Bombay. Following his Post Graduation, he rendered his services as RMO in JJ hospital Bombay and Anesthesia Consultant in various hospitals in the Kalyan region, Bombay.

Before joining SLIMS, he worked as a Teaching Faculty in NMCRH, Raichur –Karnataka, Sri Manakula Vinayagar Medical College, Pondicherry, Narayana Medical College, Nellore (AP), SLIMS Pondicherry, SSSMC&RI Chennai. The Academic qualification apart from MD anesthesia, include a PG diploma in Diabetology, Comprehensive Trauma life support (CTLS), Fellowship in pain management.

He is a recipient of FIMSA from IMSA and FICA from the Indian College of Anesthesia. He has received the Best Teacher Award from Bharat University, Chennai in September 2014 and Life Time Achievement Award ISA, ISKCON 2017, South zone. He has published 14 research papers in various National and International Journals. His areas of special interests care –ICU, Labor Analgesia, Interventional pain management, Diabetic patient care in ICU, and Podiatry (Diabetic foot care). He is the Past President of, the ISA Chapter, Puducherry.